Face It With A Puzzle
An OCD Workbook

Volume 1

Face Your Fear of Uncertainty

By Tammy LaBrake, LCSW-R

Introduction

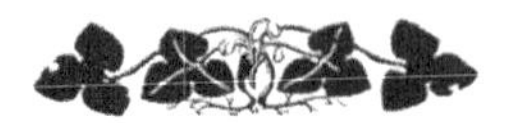

IT'S THE BELIEF THAT CERTAINTY can be obtained that gives OCD its power. If you accept how impossible it is to have certainty, you won't be so easily fooled. OCD puts doubt in your mind about whatever is precious and sacred to you. OCD lies to you and tells you there's a way to get rid of the doubt and gain certainty. Liar, liar pants on fire!

Once OCD has tricked you into thinking you can obtain certainty and be free of doubt, it's going to quickly gain more and more of your attention. OCD doesn't waste time. Give it an inch and it will take a mile. Quickly.

If you actually believe certainty is possible then OCD is going to make a promise to you. A promise that can never be fulfilled. It's going to keep lying to you about getting rid of doubt.

On the other hand, if you aren't seeking certainty, OCD has nothing to dangle in front of you. When you let go, OCD lets go. Let go or be dragged.

Practice Radical Acceptance

There's a good wolf and a bad wolf. Which one wins? The one you feed. You have a choice to feed or starve OCD. It is a choice. You can't choose your thoughts. You can't stop them. You can't control them. But you can choose how you react to them.

Whatever mystery you're trying to gain certainty over, you'll never get it. OCD will tell you to Google, ask someone for reassurance or perform a compulsion. OCD tells you THIS is how you can get certainty. So you fall for it and CHOOSE to comply rather than defy.

Perhaps you get some relief, but how long before the uncertainty creeps back? How many seconds or minutes before you're feeling doubtful and uncertain again? How long before you have to do another compulsion to get rid of the uncomfortable feeling of uncertainty?

If you choose to feed OCD it will get stronger. It's better to starve OCD so that YOU get stronger! How can you defy OCD? By accepting uncertainty. OCD can't thrive when you accept uncertainty. The more doubt you tolerate the better you get!

No matter how uncomfortable it makes you feel, shrug and say, "I don't know and might never know." The only thing that matters is right here. Right now in this moment. Be willing to find out what happens from one moment to the next.

Practice radical acceptance and surrender. Accept the "what if" as a pesky thought and focus on the present moment. Acknowledge you have a choice to feed OCD or starve it. In this moment right here, right now you have a choice. This is your chance to defy not comply.

Exposure & Response Therapy (ERP)

Seeking certainty is an unattainable goal and leads to a life not lived. The urge to seek it is so strong. It's like an addiction. ERP is about resisting this urge. Imagine what life would be like without having to do compulsions or mental acts. Free your mind. Free your life. Defy OCD.

There is a powerful way to learn how to accept uncertainty. Imagine living a life where you do absolutely nothing to obtain certainty. A life where you no longer try to control what happens. After all, a person who knows everything learns nothing.

Through the use of ERP you become desensitized to uncertainty. You repeatedly face whatever you feel uncertain about and allow the discomfort. In fact, not only do you allow the discomfort you seek it out. You look for ways to hunt it down. It's unpleasant not dangerous.

How to Use the Puzzles

These puzzles are made with words and phrases often associated with uncertainty. Some of the words reflect how uncomfortable it feels to be uncertain. How you react to the discomfort is the key. Lean into it, not away from it.

You might be so focused on solving the puzzle that you experience no anxiety, until the puzzle is solved and you suddenly realize the phrase or words are uncomfortable. So your anxiety might get triggered during or after solving a puzzle.

Words and phrases are repeated several times in this workbook. When using ERP as a treatment modality, repetition is important. You need to repeat the same exposures over and over until they have little to no effect.

Repetition breeds boredom. Your brain gets bored doing the same exposure over and over. A common mistake people make when doing ERP is that they don't do an exposure enough. So these puzzles repeatedly expose you to possible trigger words associated with uncertainty.

Hope with all your might that these puzzles trigger your anxiety. Triggering your anxiety intentionally is a good thing! Because when your anxiety is triggered you get to practice your skills. You get good at what you practice.

Not all of the puzzles will be anxiety producing. Some of them just help you practice the best way to talk to OCD. When talking to OCD it's important to say as little as possible. Don't explain or rationalize. Don't try to use logic. Just get to the shrug as quickly as possible. "Eh, whatever." ¯_(ツ)_/¯

How to Use the Exposure Worksheets

In addition to the puzzles, there are worksheets to help you create even more discomfort and uncertainty. Finding opportunities to create doubt is a very fierce effective strategy. Resisting compulsions and creating uncertainty is like Kryptonite to OCD. It deprives OCD of its powers. It's hard to be anxious when you want to be anxious.

The exposure worksheets consist of repeatedly writing anxiety-provoking words, telling a story or using stick figures to draw out your worst case scenario. Rate your anxiety at the beginning of each worksheet and at the end of the worksheet. Continue the exercise until your anxiety drops. Use additional sheets of paper if needed.

These worksheets can help you defy OCD, if used repeatedly and without any compulsive responses. If a particular word or phrase is troublesome or anxiety-provoking, then write it out on the worksheet as many times as it takes to become desensitized. Be sure to include any troublesome words of your own that you don't find in any of the puzzles.

If you like to sketch, use the worksheets to draw scenes of what you are uncertain about. You don't have to be an artist to draw. Using stick figures draw four scenes playing out your worst fear. In the first scene you have realized you can never have certainty. And then what happens next? What might happen because you can never have certainty? Draw that. And then what happens? Draw that. In the final scene, draw the worst unhappy ending you can imagine as a result of never having certainty.

While you are drawing or writing words, if you notice any anxiety, say: "Good there's my anxiety. I want this. I need the practice." Repeat what you are drawing or writing as many times needed to become desensitized.

Remember, when you are triggered, it's important to practice accepting the anxiety and agreeing with the worry. Don't try to prove OCD wrong or right. Just say, "Yup, that could happen. And if it does I'll handle it."

A Special Message From the Author: The Worksheets might not seem as rewarding as the puzzles. They are equally as important and the repetition is necessary. To make it worth your effort send me (Tammy) an email of how you used the Worksheets. Send me pictures if you like. I will return an email to you with a secret code giving you access to one of my hidden blog posts at blog.bossitback.com. This secret blog post is sure to please. If you complete your Worksheets you should get a reward! Email me about your Worksheets and I'll send you the secret code. You'll be pleasantly surprised! Email: tammy@bossitback.com

Healthy Bonus

Some of the puzzles are more difficult than others to solve. That's because there is a second purpose to this workbook. It takes dopamine to defy OCD. When you persevere and work on solving the puzzles you will produce dopamine--a neurotransmitter that provides fuel for ongoing motivation.

OCD is a big force to go up against so you need motivation and determination to persevere.

So not only do these puzzles act as an exposure exercise, and teach you how to talk to OCD, but because they are puzzles they activate healthy logical parts of your brain. It's much harder for OCD to influence you when all parts of your brain are strategically activated. Solving puzzles can make your brain a lean, mean, fighting machine.

Some of the puzzles are tough to solve. Use the tips and hints provided sparingly. Challenge your brain as much as possible!

Now that you know how to use this workbook, it's time to Face It With a Puzzle!

THE COSTS OF CERTAINTY

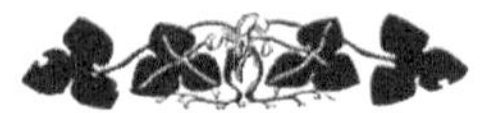

Have you noticed how much you are being robbed by trying to get certainty? Would you rather be doing something else? What does seeking certainty take you away from? Are your relationships affected? Is your productivity where you want it to be? Do you end up beating yourself up and self-loathing? Have you lost confidence in yourself? Write down what it's costing you to seek certainty:

The Benefits of Uncertainty

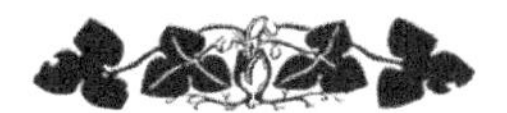

NOW THAT YOU'VE ACKNOWLEDGED what seeking certainty is costing you, let's look at what you're fighting for. If you stop seeking certainty and just accept the doubt, what will you gain? What would life look like? How would your life improve? Can you imagine how it would feel to let go of your quest for certainty?

Anyone who claims to have certainty, has stopped growing as a person. We are meant to be uncertain. If you can make uncertainty desirable, you will grow leaps and bounds. Certainty is the enemy. Don't let OCD tell you otherwise.

You've got to care about something more deeply than certainty. Write down what you are fighting for:

Words to Describe Uncertainty

The following words can be found in the diagram below reading forward, backward, up, down and diagonally. Find the words and circle them.

panic
fuzziness
danger
powerless
foolish
upheaval

dark
angst
unrest

```
O A K S X A H Q J Z E F R M Z U
M I Y Y G Q E B T W Y I P L P F
E Z G O S D P A U Y Z Y E H Q K
S E D T C B A T G B M C E Z V S
S L A W K G L D K B D A F Z D D
E E T O I X H L Z P V H F F J H
N S I I N A U O S A X F V I I S
I F J L K J P S L N O O J D W I
Z G L I G T E N L I C F T L T L
Z U F H K L R K C C A T I K F O
U T U U R I I D M F K X A O Q O
F R B E A C U H W R E G N A D F
G A W Q D L I H W L I Q G U S V
N O N Q W V U I B E G P S V X R
P X S Y T Y Y K K H S H T S A X
M T U N R E S T T A G J W C E F
```

Puzzle 1

Each of these Cryptograms is a mesage in substitution code. THE SILLY DOG might become UJD WQPPZ BVN if U is substituted for T, J for H, D for E, etc. One way to break the code is to look for repeated letters. E, T, A, O, N, R and I are the most often used letters. A single letter is usually A or I; OF, IS and IT are common 2-letter words; try THE or AND for a 3-letter group. The code is different for each Cryptogram.

k r a c

1. M vw pssjmno gsl ivre hs xlbvhb

d u

zskch. Tips: double letters (ss) are a vowel. Look for "ing." Hint: It's good to accept uncertainty but even better to look for ways to create it!

a n e h r

2. W ums sbfbo ir bsryjg kr pobfbsk

gmoa. Tip: Sometimes words with two letters are "to" or "do." Hint: Safety can never be guaranteed.

i

3. Ptte bit ptzw zvo xf pfw cb.

Tip: Double letters (tt) are a vowel. Try "the" or "and" for three letter words. Hint: You can do anything even when anxious. You can do nothing when you avoid.

Get a free book from one of Tammy's other publications by completing this survey: (Password is UnCertain) https://tjlabrake.polldaddy.com/s/face-it-with-a-puzzle-uncertainty

Puzzle 2

WORKSHEET

Use this worksheet to repeatedly write anxiety-provoking, troublesome words. Fill the page with words that trigger your anxiety about being uncertain. You are fearful about never getting to the bottom of something. Never knowing something for sure. What does uncertainty feel like? Why are you afraid of uncertainty? If there are words associated with uncertainty that trigger your anxiety, repeatedly write them down here. Note your anxiety level (on a scale of 0-7) at the beginning and end of this exercise.

Anxiety level at start _

Anxiety level at end ___

Words to Describe Uncertainty

Below is a list of scrambled words. Unscramble all the letters to reveal the words.

Tip: Look for words that begin with "un" or "dis" or end with "ess."

1. ISEYMTQU = ______________________

2. OLGOM = ______________________

3. LPEESSLSE = ______________________

4. YTSMREY = ______________________

5. EMILDMA = ______________________

6. SNNAISUESE = ______________________

7. DUFNLBEUSSOT = ______________________

8. RODSUPTIIN = ______________________

Puzzle 3

Each of these Cryptograms is a message in substitution code. THE SILLY DOG might become UJD WQPPZ BVN if U is substituted for T, J for H, D for E, etc. One way to break the code is to look for repeated letters. E, T, A, O, N, R and I are the most often used letters. A single letter is usually A or I; OF, IS and IT are common 2-letter words; try THE or AND for a 3-letter group. The code is different for each Cryptogram.

T un c e i

1. Huqa rtdgmhyqthi dlrvn vgyn hl alcghuqtf syn uywwgtqtf.

Tip: There is a vowel before and after double letters ww. Look for "ing." Hint: OCD has no power if you accept whatever happens, happens.

u e n g l

2. Dtzh wbvhdzej zh oh bjojhfvxoakv oh mjefzji tef lojc okzvjh dtvxv oxv.

Tip: Two letter words are often "is" or "as." Look for "ing." Hint: If you're trying to know something for sure then you're feeding OCD.

n g a

3. F hsskvr rukak runzpura hdi jkkefdpa, ha fa.

Tip: A single letter is often "A" or "I". Double letters in a word can be vowels or consonants. Hint: The more you resist a thought or anxiety the more they persist.

WORKSHEET

Use this worksheet to repeatedly write any troublesome words. Add your own anxiety-provoking words. Fill the page with words that trigger your anxiety about never being able to have certainty. Do this repeatedly. Let the anxiety rise and just notice it. Don't judge the anxiety as good or bad.

Anxiety level at start _

Anxiety level at end ___

The spaces between the words in the following message has been eliminated and divided into pieces. Rearrange the pieces to reconstruct the messages. The dashes indicate the number of letters in each word.

OLS OCD LFO DAY RYD AYW PRI
ITH EVE ISA

Tips: Cross out letters when you use them. EVE and RYD combined make the word EVERY and IFO combined with OLS makes the word FOOLS. Hint: OCD is a trickster!

_ _ _ _ _   _ _ _

_ _ _ _   _ _ _

_ _   _ _ _ _ _

_ _ _ _ ' _   _ _ _ .

Words to Describe Uncertainty

Below is a list of scrambled words. Unscramble all the letters to reveal the words.

Tip: Look for words that begin with "ex" or "un" or end with "y".

1. PDSEARI = ______________________

2. RHPCSCITTAAO = ______________________

3. UKRYM = ______________________

4. BYBPRLOA = ______________________

5. OHUSTEAXNI = ______________________

6. SCIIRS = ______________________

7. SANEEU = ______________________

8. REETEMX = ______________________

Puzzle 6

WORKSHEET

Write a story about the day you realized you'll never obtain certainty. Start the story with “I can never know for sure if... and as a result of never being able to get certainty this might happen..." Write the story over and over until your anxiety drops. If it's too hard to tell the whole story, then try writing a little bit of the story--a few sentences. Or, just keep writing troublesome words until they are not so troublesome. Repeat, repeat, repeat.

Anxiety level at start _

Anxiety level at end ___

Words to Describe Uncertainty

Each of the below words form a list of related words in code. When you have identified a word, use the known letters to decode the other words in the list.

1. TYVEFKPBGUHIF = UN

2. TYFUZF = UN

3. TYWYQLY = (hint: K above W)

4. TYCUVVPYFZZ = (hint: P P above V V; S S above Z Z)

5. TYBFEGUPY = (hint: C above B)

6. AUXHIF = (hint: L above H)

7. VQZZPHPIPGJ = (hint: O above Q)

8. IUBW =

Hint: Double letters often have a vowel before and after.

Puzzle 7

Words to Describe Uncertainty

To solve this puzzle, fill in the blanks below with the correct missing letter and then transfer the letter to the corresponding numbered square in the diagram below. Be careful! The puzzle is not as simple as it may first appear!

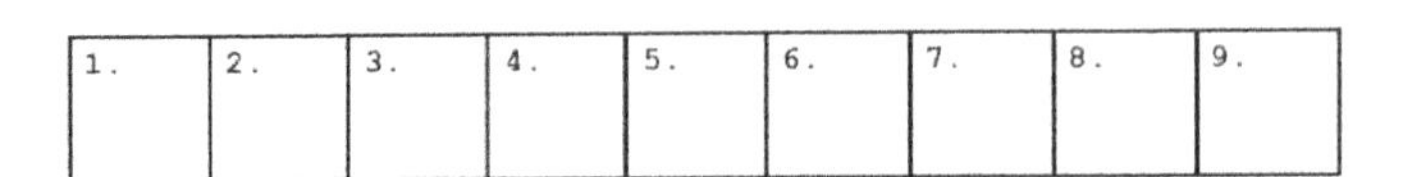

1. _ r e a d

2. s t r _ f e

3. u n r e _ t

4. m a y _ e

5. d a n g _ r

6. _ i m b o

7. c r _ s i s

8. u n _ a s e

9. _ e a r

Puzzle 8

WORKSHEET

Use this worksheet to repeatedly write any troublesome words. Use some of your own words that you haven't seen yet in a puzzle. Fill the page with words that trigger your anxiety about never being able to obtain certainty... Never knowing for sure if... While you're doing it if you note any anxiety say,"Good there's my anxiety. I want this so that I can practice living with it."

Anxiety level at start ___

Anxiety level at end ___

Words to Describe Uncertainty

Place two letters on the dashes to complete a word on the left and to begin another word on the right. For example, SE in between PLEA and VEN would complete PLEASE and begin SEVEN.

1. d i s t r u _ _ r i f e

2. s t r i _ _ a r

3. f o o l i _ _ r u g g i n g

4. d r e _ _ v e n t u r e

5. g a _ _ s t a b i l i t y

Puzzle 9

The spaces between the words in the following message have been eliminated and divided into pieces. Rearrange the pieces to reconstruct the messages. The dashes indicate the number of letters in each word.

OHWE WHOC ARES WHAT LLSO

Tips: Cross out letters after you use them. WHOC combined with ARES is WHO CARES. Hint: What you say when you are shrugging at OCD and accepting uncertainty.

_ _ _ _ _ _ , _ _

_ _ _ _ , _ _ _

_ _ _ _ _ .

Puzzle 10

WORKSHEET

Instead of telling the story, you can draw out the story. Using stick figures draw four scenes playing out your worst fear. In the first scene you realize you'll never know for sure about... And then what happens next? Draw that. And then what happens? Draw that. In the final scene, draw the worst unhappy ending as a result of never having certainty. Repeat this until the drawing no longer bothers you.

Anxiety level at start __

Anxiety level at end ___

Words to Describe Uncertainty

four
Rearrange and distribute the ~~five~~ letters accompanying each row so that you form a larger common word.

The typo above doesn't mean toss out the page and start over!

1. s e e n : __ u s p __ __ s __

2. b e e n : t u r __ u l __ __ c __

3. a c i d : __ __ s __ o u r __ g e

4. e v e n : __ a g u __ __ __ s s

5. f i n e : __ u z z __ __ __ s s

Puzzle 11

Each of these Cryptograms is a message in substitution code. THE SILLY DOG might become UJD WQPPZ BVN if U is substituted for T, J for H, D for E, etc. One way to break the code is to look for repeated letters. E, T, A, O, N, R and I are the most often used letters. A single letter is usually A or I; OF, IS and IT are common 2-letter words; try THE or AND for a 3-letter group. <u>The code is different for each Cryptogram</u>.

s u t o

1. Jatv defmbjcteju fkdin smce

me b

vksmjatel pcn acggmev.

Tip: There is a vowel before and after double letters. Hint: When OCD says this it's important to say, "It's unpleasant but I can handle it."

2. L ya jqqflbd nqk oyuh zq xkiyzi tqvpz.

Hint: You already know this is how you get stronger.

h

3. C xte edodg mv devpnu iv agdodei

a

utgf.

Hint: You already know this to be the truth.

Puzzle 12

WORKSHEET

As before, using stick figures draw four scenes playing out your worst fear about never obtaining certainty about...

When you become desensitized to this story, draw a new story.

Anxiety level at start ___

Anxiety level at end ___

The below messages are in a number code based on how text messages are formed on a 'flip phone'. Each number represents one of the letters shown on the picture of the phone to the left. You must decide which one. A number is not necessarily the same letter each time.

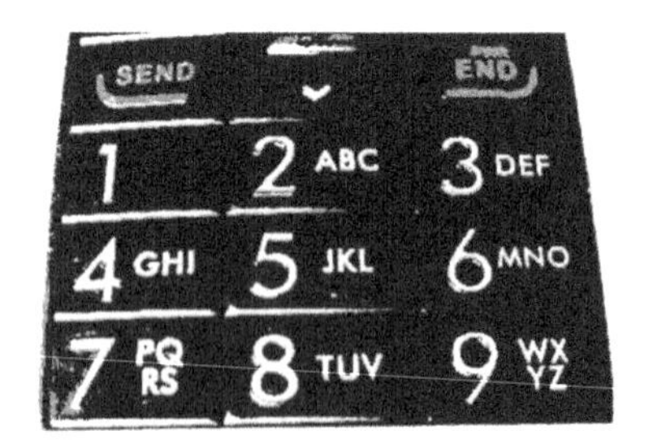

Two letter word 46: GHI MNO could be GO or IN

1. 4 24733 9484 968, 623.

Hint: Figure out single words first. Eliminate rare letters like X Z. Tip: It never pays to argue or use logic with OCD.

om 100 le

2. 46 2 7666 3855 63 100 736753, 6678 63 8436 968536'8 96779 22688 8447.

Hint: Figure out single, double lettered words then contractions. Tip: If other people don't have to worry about this than neither do you.

Puzzle 13

Words to Describe Uncertainty

Insert a different letter of the alphabet into each of the 26 empty boxes to form words reading across. The letter you insert may be at the beginning, the end or the middle of the word. Each letter of the alphabet will be used only once. Cross off each letter in the list as you use it. All the letters in each row are not necessarily used in forming the word.

Example: In the first row, we have inserted the letter Z to form the word DAZED

A B C D E F G H I J K L M N O P Q R S T U V W X Y ~~Z~~

D	R	K	W	D	A	**Z**	E	D	R	A	A	I	dazed
Y	A	C	I	F	F	**Y**	H	P	N	N	H	I	iffy
N	Z	Z	S	U	S		E	N	S	E	X	R	
K	S	I	R	I	S		Y	T	P	I	S	H	
S	N	J	J	X	Z		E	A	R	Z	R	M	
A	U	N	C	E	R		A	I	N	P	D	Q	
E	V	A	M	B	I		U	I	T	Y	O	L	
I	M	Y	S	T	I		U	E	Q	H	Q	J	
M	F	D	P	R	O		A	B	L	Y	C	H	
C	O	N	C	E	R		J	Q	I	M	K	I	
B	G	U	E	S	S		O	R	K	E	K	A	
A	R	M	U	N	R		S	T	I	G	S	O	
G	G	L	E	P	W		O	U	B	T	S	F	
P	C	O	N	F	U		I	O	N	K	C	T	
U	S	L	E	E	P		E	S	S	X	C	J	
G	M	I	S	G	I		I	N	G	S	E	W	
O	V	U	I	G	N		R	A	N	C	E	Z	
Y	P	T	U	R	B		L	E	N	C	E	B	
B	T	U	R	M	O		L	U	C	T	Z	C	
M	V	V	Q	S	H		K	Y	J	P	Q	U	
P	E	R	P	L	E		E	D	D	H	S	L	
J	S	H	D	P	N		Y	S	T	E	R	Y	
F	O	O	L	I	S		Q	Y	U	W	F	G	
L	M	L	R	E	Z		I	T	T	E	R	S	
U	K	I	N	S	E		U	R	I	T	Y	I	
P	L	D	I	S	A		R	A	Y	G	R	U	

Puzzle 14

WORKSHEET

Write a story about the day you realized you'll never obtain certainty... Start the story with “I can never know for sure if... as a result of never being able to get certainty this might happen..." Write the story over and over until your anxiety drops. If it's too hard to tell the whole story, then try writing a little bit of the story--a few sentences. Or, just keep writing troublesome words until they are not so troublesome. Repeat, repeat, repeat.

Anxiety level at start ______

Anxiety level at end ___

The spaces between the words in the following message has been eliminated and divided into pieces. Rearrange the pieces to reconstruct the messages. The dashes indicate the number of letters in each word.

TOP 'TME RDO ESN ANS FEA

Hint: Just because you feel this it doesn't mean you shouldn't keep going.

_ _ _ _   _ _ _ _ _ '_

_ _ _ _   _ _ _ _ .

Puzzle 15

Words to Describe Uncertainty

Below is a list of scrambled words. Unscramble all the letters to reveal the words.

Tips: Look for words that begin with "dis" or "un" or end with "ness" or "ence"

1. ADAIYRSR = ______________________

2. UTLRCBNUEE = ______________________

3. ERESPRSSU = ______________________

4. EDSNINIEEISVSC = ______________________

5. NGAGNIG = ______________________

6. TISJRTE = ______________________

7. ENRONCNC = ______________________

8. UDTOB = ______________________

Puzzle 16

WORKSHEET

Use this page to repeatedly write any troublesome words. Fill the page with words that trigger your anxiety about living with uncertainty for the rest of your life. While you're doing it if you note any anxiety say, "Good there's my anxiety. I want this so that I can practice being with it."

Anxiety level at start __________

Anxiety level at end ___

Words to Describe Uncertainty

Each of the below words form a list of related words in code. When you have identified a word, use the known letters to decode the other words in the list.

1. TDGFCXCH = ____________________

2. BOYJTDNOKV = ____________________

3. TVGCDDOVFYY = ____________________

4. YHFFDHFYY = ____________________

5. ACJOVFYY = ____________________

6. NFVYOKV = ____________________

7. UTFYYAKJZ = ____________________

8. CVUTOYG = ____________________

Tips: Look for words that begin with "dis" or "un" or end with "tion" or "ess"

Puzzle 17

Words to Describe Uncertainty

To solve this puzzle, fill in the blanks below with the correct missing letter and then transfer the letter to the corresponding numbered square in the diagram below. Be careful! The puzzle is not as simple as it may first appear!

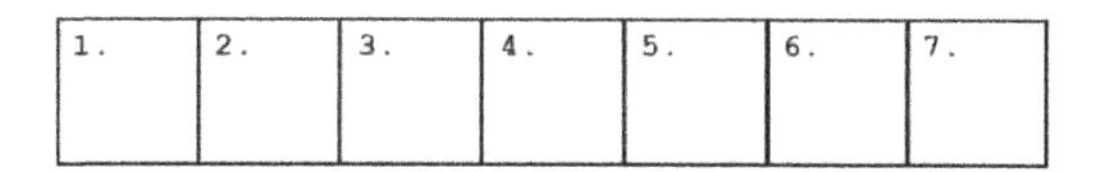

1. _ a y b e

2. w o r r _

3. u n e a _ e

4. s _ r i f e

5. u n s u r _

6. d a _ k

7. m u r k _

Puzzle 18

WORKSHEET

Your Choice: Either write troublesome words, or write a "once upon a time" story about waking up with no certainty about anything. If you're not feeling much anxiety, make sure you're not avoiding any words or stories.

Anxiety level at start ______

Anxiety level at end ___

The below messages are in a number code based on how text messages are formed on a 'flip phone'. Each number represents one of the letters shown on the picture of the phone to the left. You must decide which one. A number is not necessarily the same letter each time.

SEND
END
1
2 ABC
3 DEF
4 GHI
5 JKL
6 MNO
7 PQ RS
8 TUV
9 WX YZ

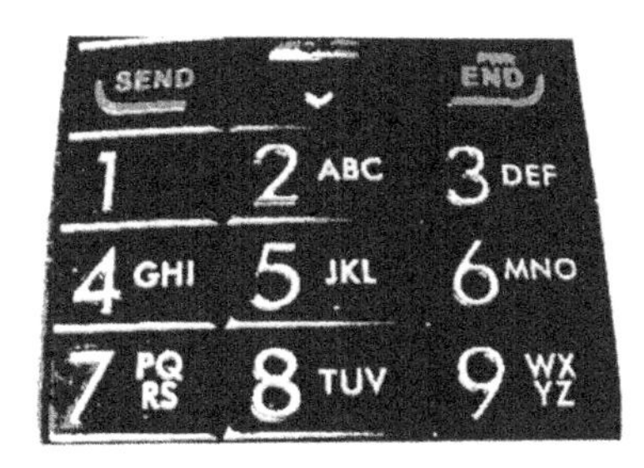

Tips: Figure out contractions first, then 2 letter words. Look for word parts like the ending "ing."

1. 4'3 728437 3335 843 3327.

Hint: It's better to feel this than live a life avoiding it.

2. 4'6 46464 8692737 843 2694389, 668 2929.

Hint: OCD only remains strong until you stop running from it. Learn how to experience it.

Puzzle 19

The spaces between the words in the following message has been eliminated and divided into pieces. Rearrange the pieces to reconstruct the messages. The dashes indicate the number of letters in each word.

NDG LTH EFE OFO RIT FEE ARA

Hint: You already know this is important. Everything you ever wanted is on the other side of it.

_ _ _ _ _ _ _

_ _ _ _ _ _ _

_ _ _ _ _ _ _ .

Puzzle 20

WORKSHEET

Using stick figures draw four scenes playing out your worst fear. In the first scene you realize you'll never know for sure about... And then what happens next? Draw that. And then what happens? Draw that. In the final scene, draw the worst unhappy ending as a result of never having certainty. Repeat this until you're bored drawing it. The whole point of repeating an exposure over and over is to get bored!

Anxiety level at start _____

Anxiety level at end ___

Each of these Cryptograms is a message in substitution code. THE SILLY DOG might become UJD WQPPZ BVN if U is substituted for T, J for H, D for E, etc. One way to break the code is to look for repeated letters. E, T, A, O, N, R and I are the most often used letters. A single letter is usually A or I; OF, IS and IT are common 2-letter words; try THE or AND for a 3-letter group. The code is different for each Cryptogram.

1. N lpg's fgpk vph uahx sers senu nu waus PQL.

f r h

Tip: Figure out the one and two letter words first. Think, what abbreviation would be capitalized? Hint: Everybody gets weird thoughts. It's your reaction to them that causes the problem.

2. A'n udyjcu ydgc yjc uavg dpn pctcu gpkm.

a t r k

Hint: Isn't it better to live with uncertainty than spend a lifetime trying to get what can't be gotten?

3. Dvhcm hfa'om otils FBK.

e i h

Hint: It's better to not argue. Just nod and play along.

Puzzle 21

Words to Describe Uncertainty

The following words can be found in the diagram below reading forward, backward, up, down and diagonally. Find the words and circle them.

sleepless
unrest
chaos
inadequacy
dark
guesswork

random
limbo
tumult
vagueness
angst
lack

```
S C H A O S T R C D A R K H F N
P S R D X Y I T E X J I W B Y S
F M A R P Z B F K J V C D M L E
G U N R E S T L S R A L V E X I
U K D D R O B A X X B V E D N N
E N O T N O Y X X T A P B T G A
S F M M Y X M K S K L U W U L D
S C I Y C G V E S E C Z S M I E
W P S F D R D S S B L D C U M Q
O R I O Q A E S F B B Y L L B U
R V U O E N S Q K O V N O T O A
K N C H E G T F Y W G J A J B C
I X S U O S Z T M L O G Z T Z Y
P E G O L T R C Z T J T Z I P G
R A P P T Y N L M M E Y X T F W
V M F M Q T Y I L A C K W X B G
```

Puzzle 22

WORKSHEET

Write a story about the day you realized you'll never obtain certainty... Start the story with “I can never know for sure if... as a result of never being able to get certainty this might happen..." If your anxiety is remaining high, consider reading your story out loud, using an accent.

Anxiety level at start _____

Anxiety level at end ____

Words to Describe Uncertainty

Rearrange and distribute the five letters accompanying each row so that you form a larger common word.

1. none: c __ __ s __ q u e __ c e s

2. need: u __ s __ t t l __ __

3. days: __ i __ __ r r a __

4. base: u n __ t __ __ l __

5. nine: u __ h a p p __ __ __ s s

Get a free book by completing this survey:
https://tjlabrake.polldaddy.com/s/face-it-with-a-puzzle-uncertainty
Password is UnCertain

Puzzle 23

Words to Describe Uncertainty

Below is a list of scrambled words. Unscramble all the letters to reveal the words.

Tip: Look for words that begin with "un" or end with "ing" or "ness"

1. PIEBLTCDRUENA = ______________________

2. IEAITNGVYT = ______________________

3. OKUGSWRSE = ______________________

4. NATGS = ______________________

5. VEGUASESN = ______________________

6. SVUSNEGAE = ______________________

7. AGNIGGN = ______________________

8. ADNMOR = ______________________

Puzzle 24

WORKSHEET

Your Method of Choice: Either write troublesome words, write a "never knowing for sure about..." story, or use stick figures to draw out four horror scenes about never feeling certain about... Of the three methods are you choosing the easiest all the time? Work your way up to the hardest method. It's important to build momentum. Remember what you're fighting for.

Anxiety level at start _____

Anxiety level at end ___

Words to Describe Uncertainty

Below is a list of scrambled words. Unscramble all the letters to reveal the words.

Tip: Look for words that start with "in" or "dis" or end with "tion" or "y"

1. BYTTIIILNSA = ______________________

2. OPYSTBISIIL = ______________________

3. EDSBEIILF = ______________________

4. AINUOSXETH = ______________________

5. SYYTERM = ______________________

6. ODENIITPATR = ______________________

7. ESETNUDTL = ______________________

8. DSIUTTSR = ______________________

Puzzle 25

The following words can be found in the diagram below reading forward, backward, up, down and diagonally. Find the words and circle them.

lack	unknown
unrest	unrest
panic	unease
wariness	disbelief
dread	fret
probably	dark

U	W	D	O	U	D	Y	L	B	A	B	O	R	P	K	Y
J	N	K	G	Y	R	Q	I	L	I	U	F	Z	D	Z	L
S	P	K	Y	G	D	U	X	H	U	N	R	E	S	T	A
M	V	F	N	J	Y	T	D	C	D	R	C	L	O	J	C
K	F	Z	S	O	R	H	X	R	L	E	X	J	A	V	K
Q	E	P	N	M	W	C	J	R	L	S	I	K	P	K	O
S	W	C	B	G	I	N	A	Z	A	T	I	X	R	T	U
A	U	P	R	Z	F	F	L	H	O	C	T	W	N	I	H
B	A	E	E	B	K	N	S	C	K	N	K	H	F	E	D
D	B	F	Z	R	X	Y	X	S	C	K	F	R	N	Y	R
A	O	A	H	W	C	I	A	H	E	K	L	V	M	V	E
R	J	X	C	O	C	E	T	C	I	N	A	P	B	W	A
K	R	A	T	T	K	Y	L	X	X	Z	I	Y	E	V	D
A	M	V	I	W	F	R	E	T	G	D	J	R	C	M	H
F	A	J	J	U	U	N	E	A	S	E	K	G	A	L	K
Z	F	V	Y	Q	F	E	I	L	E	B	S	I	D	W	S

Puzzle 26

WORKSHEET

If you've gotten used to the words and images associated with living with uncertainty, it's time to take bigger steps. Are there any people, places or things you've been avoiding because of feeling uncertain? Make a list of them. If you were to stop avoiding, rate them in terms of most anxiety- provoking to least. Starting with the least anxiety-provoking trigger, it's time to stop avoiding and live your life. Begin your gradual mission to face whatever you're avoiding. It might be hard. But, it's your path to freedom.

Anxiety level at start ____

Anxiety level at end ___

To receive a free book please complete this survey:
https://tjlabrake.polldaddy.com/s/face-it-with-a-puzzle-uncertainty Password is UnCertain.

In Summary

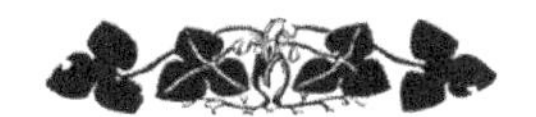

Tips to Remember

- Repetition breeds boredom.
- Confront your fear repeatedly and you will get bored!
- Avoidance breeds anxiety.
- You can't heal what you won't feel.
- Face your fears and feel the anxiety.
- Agree with OCD, don't argue with it.
- Talk to OCD as if uncertainty doesn't matter to you.
- Repeatedly confront trigger words, stories and drawings.
- Make sure you repeatedly do it.
- When you become desensitized to words move on to real life situations.
- If you only confront a feared situation sporadically, it'll likely be traumatic.
- Confront your fears repeatedly. And accelerate. Build momentum.

ABOUT THE AUTHOR

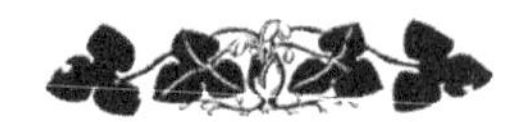

- Tammy LaBrake, is a licensed Clinical Social Worker (LCSW) and founder of a private practice in New York known as, Boss It Back® which is dedicated to the treatment of OCD.

- As an unorthodox thinker, she values cutting edge developments and enjoys using creativity in her practice.

- Tammy agrees with the evidence-based effectiveness of Exposure & Response (ERP)therapy in the treatment of OCD. It's important to address OCD as soon as possible and so she created a series of OCD puzzle books to make ERP exercises readily available.

- Tammy is a member of the International OCD Foundation and is a graduate of the Foundation's Behavior Training Therapy Institute.

- She is the author of other publications such as the innovative OCD Coloring Book. Go to Amazon and check out her reviews!

- For more ideas on ERP, visit blog.bossitback.com and search Exposure & Response Prevention.

- If you would like to receive tips on a regular basis, please join Tammy's free email list at: OCDstrategies.com

- You can also follow Tammy on Twitter at: @tjlabrake or Facebook (Search: Free Your Life. Free Your Mind. Defy OCD.)

Best wishes in your Boss it Back endeavors! You're stronger than you know!

Don't forget to email Tammy about your Worksheets (tammy@bossitback.com) and get your secret code to unlock a hidden blog post. Your efforts will be rewarded with a surprise! Also, get a free book by completing this survey: https://tjlabrake.polldaddy.com/s/face-it-with-a-puzzle-uncertainty. Password is UnCertain.

ANSWER KEY

Puzzle 1

O	A	K	S	X	A	H	Q	J	Z	E	F	R	M	Z	U
M	I	Y	Y	G	Q	E	B	T	W	Y	I	P	L	P	F
E	Z	G	O	S	D	P	A	U	Y	Z	Y	E	H	Q	K
S	E	D	T	C	B	A	T	G	B	M	C	E	Z	V	S
S	L	A	W	K	G	L	D	K	B	D	A	F	Z	D	D
E	E	T	O	I	X	H	L	Z	P	V	H	F	F	J	H
N	S	I	I	N	A	U	O	S	A	X	F	V	I	I	S
I	F	J	L	K	J	P	S	L	N	O	O	J	D	W	I
Z	G	L	I	G	T	E	N	L	I	C	F	T	L	T	L
Z	U	F	H	K	L	R	K	C	C	A	T	I	K	F	O
U	T	U	U	R	I	I	D	M	F	K	X	A	O	Q	O
F	R	B	E	A	C	U	H	W	R	E	G	N	A	D	F
G	A	W	Q	D	L	I	H	W	L	I	Q	G	U	S	V
N	O	N	Q	W	V	U	I	B	E	G	P	S	V	X	R
P	X	S	Y	T	Y	Y	K	K	H	S	H	T	S	A	X
M	T	U	N	R	E	S	T	T	A	G	J	W	C	E	F

Puzzle 2

1. M vw pssjmno gsl ivre hs xlbvhb zskch.

   I am looking for ways to create doubt.

2. W ums sbfbo ir bsryjg kr pobfbsk gmoa.

   I can never do enough to prevent harm.

3. Ptte bit ptzw zvo xf pfw cb.

   Feel the fear and go for it.

Puzzle 3

1. ISEYMTQU - **MYSTIQUE**
2. OLGOM - **GLOOM**
3. LPEESSLSE - **SLEEPLESS**
4. YTSMREY = **MYSTERY**
5. EMILDMA = **DILEMMA**
6. SNNAISUESE = **UNEASINESS**
7. DUFNLBEUSSOT - **DOUBTFULNESS**
8. RODSUPTIIN - **DISRUPTION**

Puzzle 4

1. Huqa rtdqmhyqthi dlrvn vqyn hi alcqhuqtf syn uywwqtqtf.

   This uncertainty could lead to something bad happening.

2. Dtzh wbvhdzej zh oh bjojhfvxoakv oh mjefzji tef lojc okzvjh dtvxv oxv.

   This question is as unanswerable as knowing how many aliens there are.

3. F hsskvr rukak runzpura hdi jkkefdpa, ha fa.

   I accept these thoughts and feelings, as is.

ANSWER KEY

Puzzle 5

e v e r y d a y
w i t h o c d
i s a p r i l
f o o l 's d a y .

Puzzle 6

1. PDSEARI = DESPAIR
2. RHPCSCITTAAO = CATASTROPHIC
3. UKRYM = MURKY
4. BYBPRLOA = PROBABLY
5. OHUSTEAXNI = EXHAUSTION
6. SCIIRS = CRISIS
7. SANEEU = UNEASE
8. REETEMX = EXTREME

Puzzle 7

1. TYVEFKPBGUHIF UNPREDICTABLE
2. TYFUZF = UNEASE
3. TYWYQLY = UNKNOWN
4. TYCUVVPYFZZ = UNHAPPINESS
5. TYBFEGUPY = UNCERTAIN
6. AUXHIF = GAMBLE
7. VQZZPHPIPGJ = POSSIBILITY
8. IUBW = LACK

Puzzle 8

| d | i | s | b | e | l | i | e | f |

1. d r e a d
2. s t r i f e
3. u n r e s t
4. m a y b e
5. d a n g e r
6. l i m b o
7. c r i s i s
8. u n e a s e
9. f e a r

ANSWER KEY

Puzzle 9

1. d i s t r u s t r i f e
2. s t r i f e a r
3. f o o l i s h r u g g i n g
4. d r e a d v e n t u r e
5. g a i n s t a b i l i t y

Puzzle 10

o h w e l l , s o
w h a t , w h o
c a r e s .

Puzzle 11

1. s e e n : s u s p e n s e
2. b e e n : t u r p u l e n c e
3. a c i d : d i s c o u r a g e
4. e v e n : v a g u e n e s s
5. f i n e : f u z z i n e s s

Puzzle 12

1. Jatv detmbjcteju tkdin smce vksmjatel pcn acggmev.

   This uncertainty could mean something bad happens.

2. L ya jqqflbd nqk oyuh zq xkiyzi tqvpz.

   I am looking for ways to create doubt.

3. C xte edodg mv devpnu iv agdodei utgf.

   I can never do enough to prevent harm.

ANSWER KEY

Puzzle 13

1. 4 24733 9484 968, 623.

   I agree with you, 100%.

2. 46 2 7666 3855 63 100 736753, 6678 63 8436 968536'8 96779 22688 8447.

   In a room full of 100 people, most of them wouldn't worry about this.

Puzzle 14

D	R	K	W	D	A	**Z**	E	D	R	A	A	I
Y	A	C	I	F	F	Y	H	P	N	N	H	T
N	Z	Z	B	U	S	P	E	N	S	E	X	R
K	S	I	R	I	S	K	Y	T	P	I	S	H
S	N	J	J	X	Z	F	E	A	R	Z	R	M
A	U	N	C	E	R	T	A	I	N	P	D	Q
E	V	A	M	B	I	G	U	I	T	Y	O	L
I	M	Y	S	T	I	Q	U	E	Q	H	Q	J
M	F	D	P	R	O	B	A	B	L	Y	C	H
C	O	N	C	E	R	N	J	Q	I	M	K	I
B	G	U	E	S	S	W	O	R	K	E	K	A
A	R	M	U	N	R	E	S	T	I	G	S	O
G	G	L	E	P	W	D	O	U	B	T	S	F
P	C	O	N	F	U	S	I	O	N	K	C	T
U	S	L	E	E	P	L	E	S	S	X	C	J
G	M	I	S	G	I	V	I	N	G	S	E	W
O	V	U	I	G	N	O	K	A	N	C	E	Z
Y	P	T	U	R	B	U	L	E	N	C	E	B
B	T	U	R	M	O	I	L	U	C	T	Z	C
M	V	V	Q	S	H	A	K	Y	J	P	Q	U
P	E	R	P	L	E	X	E	D	D	H	S	L
J	S	H	D	P	N	M	Y	S	T	E	R	Y
F	O	O	L	I	S	H	Q	Y	U	W	F	G
L	M	L	R	E	Z	J	I	T	T	E	R	S
U	K	I	N	S	E	C	U	R	I	T	Y	I
P	L	D	T	S	A	R	R	A	Y	G	R	U

Puzzle 15

t e a r d o e s n 't
m e a n s t o p .

Puzzle 16

1. ADAIYRSR = **DISARRAY**
2. UTLRCBNUEE = **TURBULENCE**
3. ERESPRSSU = **PRESSURES**
4. EDSNINIEEISVSC **INDECISIVENESS**
5. NGAGNIC = **NAGGING**
6. TISJRTE = **JITTERS**
7. ENROCNC = **CONCERN**
8. UDTOB = **DOUBT**

ANSWER KEY

Puzzle 17

1. TDGFCXCH UPHEAVAL
2. BOYJTDNOKV = DISRUPTION
3. TVGCDDOVFYY = UNHAPPINESS
4. YHFFDHFYY = SLEEPLESS
5. ACJOVFYY = WARINESS
6. NFVYOKV TENSION
7. UTFYYAKJZ = GUESSWORK
8. CVUTOYG = ANGUISH

Puzzle 18

m	y	s	t	e	r	y

1. m a y b e
2. w o r r y
3. u n e a s e
4. s t r i f e
5. u n s u r e
6. d a r k
7. m u r k y

Puzzle 19

1. 4'3 728437 3335 843 3327.

   I'd rather feel the fear.

2. 4'6 46464 8692737 843 2694389, 668 2929.

   I'm going towards the anxiety, not away.

Puzzle 20

f e e l   t h e

f e a r   a n d

g o   f o r   i t .

Answer Key

Puzzle 21

1. N lpg's tgpk vph uahx sers senu nu waus PQL.

   I don't know for sure that this is just OCD.

2. A'n udyjcu ydgc yjc uavg dpn pctcu gpkm.

   I'd rather take the risk and never know.

3. Dvhcm hta'om otils FBK.

   Maybe you're right OCD.

Puzzle 22

```
S C H A O S T R C D A R K H F N
P S R D X Y I T E X J I W B Y S
F M A R P Z B F K J V C D M L E
G U N R E S T L S R A L V E X I
U K D D R O B A X X B V E D N N
E N O T N O Y X X T A F B T G A
S F M M Y X M K S K L U W U L D
S C I Y C G V E S E C Z S M I E
W P S F D R D S S B L D C U M Q
O R I O Q A E S F B B Y L L B U
R V U O E N S Q K O V N O T O A
K N C H E G T F Y W G J A J B C
I X S U O S Z T M L O G Z T Z Y
P E G O L T R C Z T J T Z I P G
R A P P T Y N L M M E Y X T F W
V M F M Q T Y I L A C K W X B G
```

Puzzle 23

1. none: c o n s e q u e n c e s
2. need: u n s e t t l i n g
3. days: d i s a r r a y
4. base: u n s t a b l e
5. nine: u n h a p p i n e s s

Puzzle 24

1. PIEBLTCDRUENA UNPREDICTABLE
2. IEAITNGVYT = NEGATIVITY
3. OKUGSWRSE = GUESSWORK
4. NATGS = ANGST
5. VEGUASESN = VAGUENESS
6. SVUSNEGAE = VAGUENESS
7. AGNIGGN = NAGGING
8. ADNMOR = RANDOM

Answer Key

Puzzle 25

1. BYTTIIILNSA = **INSTABILITY**
2. OPYSTBISIIL = **POSSIBILITY**
3. EDSBEIILF = **DISBELIEF**
4. AINUOSXETH = **EXHAUSTION**
5. SYYTERM = **MYSTERY**
6. ODENIITPATR = **TREPIDATION**
7. ESETNUDTL = **UNSETTLED**
8. DSIUTTSR = **DISTRUST**

Puzzle 26

```
U W D O U D Y L B A B O R P K Y
J N K G Y R Q I L I U F Z D Z L
S P K Y G D U X H U N R E S T A
M V F N J Y T D C D R C L O J C
K F Z S O R H X R L E X J A V K
Q E P N M W C J R L S I K P K O
S W C B G I N A Z A T I X R T U
A U P R Z F F L H O C T W N I H
B A E E B K N S C K N K H F E D
D B F Z R X Y X S C K F R N Y R
A O A H W C I A H E K L V M V E
R J X C O C E T C I N A P B W A
K R A T T K Y L X X Z I Y E V D
A M V I W F R E T G D J R C M H
F A J J U U N E A S E K C A L K
Z F V Y Q F E I L E B S I D W S
```

This publication is part of a series of products and publications. For more information, please visit Tammy LaBrake's website at OCDstrategies.com

BossitBack® Productions

 This workbook is not intended to provide exact details or advice and is for informational purposes only. The information in this workbook is not intended as a substitute for consultation with health care professionals. It is recommended that the user of this workbook have basic knowledge of Exposure & Response Prevention (ERP) therapy.

The author reserves the right to make any changes necessary to maintain the integrity of the information held within. This workbook is not presented as legal, accounting or counseling advice. Each individual's health concerns should be evaluated by a qualified professional.

ISBN 978-0-9983597-2-4

Made in the USA
Coppell, TX
15 December 2019